Ten – Nine – Twenty One
More of Jesus, Less of Me
Forty Day Challenge

Ten – Nine – Twenty One

Ten – Nine – Twenty One
More of Jesus, Less of Me
Forty Day Challenge

Terri Flynn

Scriptures quotations taken from www.biblegateway.com

Scripture quotations marked ESV are from The Holy Bible, English Standard Version® copyright © 2001 by Crossway, a publishing ministry of Good News Publishers. Used by permission.

Scripture quotations marked KJV are taken from the King James Version of the Bible, Public domain.

Scripture quotations marked NIV are from the Holy Bible, New International Version. Copyright © 1973, 1978, 1884, International Bible Society. Used by permission.

The Master Cleanser published in 1976 Stanley Burroughs published.

An application to register this book for cataloging has been submitted to the Library of Congress.

ISBN- 13: 978-1518888076 Soft cover
ISBN- 10: 1518888070 E-Book
https://www.createspace.com/5838774

Dedication

I dedicate this book to my Lord and Savior. I want to thank You, Lord, for bringing Rose and Frank in to my life, and for giving me the opportunity to save a life. I have asked myself why You would give us two kidneys if we only needed one; I am certain now that You gave us one to keep and one to give away.

Contents

Preface

This is my testimony of how God ordained my steps as a young child and brought two little girls together to save a man's life. I am certain that God ordains every step we take. We all have a journey with a purpose and destiny that God has planned for us. My journey began when my family moved to a new neighborhood in Kingston, New York where I met my best friend Rose. Our paths crossed when God placed me in a home across the field from hers. I was 4 years old and she was 5. As we grew, we were inseparable sisters at heart. We had no idea what God had planned for us. Proverbs 20:24, "Man's steps are ordained by the Lord, how then can man understand His way?"

As I look back, I can see God's hand working in my life. God is always working things together for good, but not just for my good. Sometimes we are part of His working things together for someone else's good, but we don't know it yet. When I was around 8 or 9 years old God started whispering in to my spirt that I would one day give Rose a kidney. I was not sure why I was having this thought which just came out of nowhere. The thought that I would give Rose a kidney would come and go throughout the years. I would ponder on it for a while but I kept it to myself I never told anyone about it. I was afraid people would think that I was weird since Rose didn't need a kidney. I know now that God was preparing me for a journey later on in my life. Romans 8:28, "And we know that in all things God works for the good of those who love him, who have been called according to His purpose."

Many years had passed and a thousand miles separated us but our friendship remained strong, and the thought of giving up a kidney faded until June 2012. Then the Holy Spirit started speaking to me again about giving Rose a kidney. I could not get it out of my mind for the entire month of June. I started praying and asking God for guidance and wisdom. Why was I having these thoughts? What did they mean? Was Rose sick and unware of it? I needed God's direction. This thought was too strong to be nothing. One thing I've found out in life is that when I am following God's will and obeying His voice He will give me confirmation.

Then one Friday evening the first confirmation came. Rose called to give me the news that her husband Frank was in renal failure and needed a kidney. I was blown away, I was speechless. I quickly hung up with her and prayed asking God if He really wanted me to donate my kidney. I don't believe there are coincidences. Coincidences are really God's hand in our life. It is God speaking to us and giving us direction and confirmation. Proverbs 16:33, *"We toss the coin, but it is the Lord who controls its decision."*

The next day my husband Sean and I are in the car with our daughters and out of the blue our girls started talking about donating a kidney. I quietly laugh inside and said "Lord, You have got to be kidding." So my family and I had a lengthy discussion about kidney donation. I asked Sean if he would consider donating a kidney and he replied "yes I would." Up to this point I had still not told my family or anyone about Frank or what I though God was telling me to do. I continued to pray asking God for guidance and wisdom. I did not want to say it out loud if God was not telling me to do it. Then I did some research and I watched a YouTube video to see what the surgery entailed. Then Sunday night I told Sean what I believed God was telling me to do. Sean immediately agreed that I should donate my kidney to Frank. So we were in agreement. That was my second confirmation.

Rose and Frank were together for 25 years before they got married in 2011. The Bible tells us that marriage bonds us together as one. Mark 10: 8 says, *"The two will become one. So they are no longer two, but one."* For that reason I would essentially be giving Rose a kidney, when I gave my kidney to Frank. This is because Frank and Rose are one flesh since they are married.

I called Rose to tell her what God had been preparing me to do and we both knew it was a miracle orchestrated by God. So I started undergoing various medical tests to determine if I was a match, and I was a match. That was my third confirmation. Next we needed to see if I was healthy enough to donate the organ responsible for filtering the body's blood; after many test the doctors conclude I was in good health. However, I was a little overweight to donate an organ without potentially endangering my own health. So I would need to lose at least 19 pounds, before they would consider me as a candidate. They will only transplant individuals within the normal weight BMI. Recognizing I could make a meaningful change in Frank's personal health was really a great motivator to get the weight off. I knew it was time for me to get serious. I turned to God and asked for His help since losing weigh over the past eight years has been a struggle for me. Then I came up with the weight loss program Ten – Nine – Twenty One; that helped me loss the weight with out starving myself. I lost 27 pounds in 40 days, enough for me to be eligible to donate. I had no doubt that God's hand was arranging my steps for many years; preparing me for such a time as this.

It was happening, I was donating a kidney to Frank. The transplant surgery took place July 6th, 2015 and it was successful. Frank and I are both recovering well; the doctors are very pleased. God just amazes me how He is in every little detail. I was told before the surgery to expect a lot of pain. Because the spleen, stomach, and intestine lie near the kidney, they needed to be moved in order to remove the kidney and this causes a lot of pain after the surgery as they settle back into place. The surgery is done by hand-assisted laparoscopy using a two smaller incision in the abdomen and a vertical incision near the belly button through which a hand is inserted to hold and then remove the kidney. After the surgery I found out that my left kidney, the one I donated, had extra-long arteries. God knew before I was born that I would one day need extra-long arteries on my left kidney. Because my arties where extra-long the incision was made just below my bra line instead of near the belly bottom as a result none of the other organs needed to be moved out of the way. Most people need to take pain medicine at home for 3-4 weeks following the surgery because of the pain. However, the only pain I experienced was a soreness in my abdomen; it felt like I did too many crunches. So I was done taking the pain medicine by the time I was released from the hospital 4 days later. Psalm 139:13 tells us, "You are the one who created my innermost parts; You knit me together."

I just stand in awe of Jesus, He is my healer. I am so grateful God gave me the opportunity to give the gift of life. I don't consider myself a hero for what I did and I don't want any of the credit. I want people to look at Jesus. It's the strength that He's given me that enabled me to do this. I want all the glory to be directed at Him not me.

Terri Flynn

Chapter 1

Making a Change

I have spent most of my life struggling with eating properly, stuck in a constant cycle of indulging, then gaining weight, starving myself and then losing weight. I have repeated this cycle over and over again for 40 plus years. Long before I was a teenager I have been worried about being fat, which resulted in some really unhealthy dieting habits; very often not eating at all. My friend Patty and I both had older brother and they would always tease us and call us fat. From that point on how I saw myself and how much I weight has always been an ongoing struggle for me. Even when I was at my thinnest I would still look in the mirror and think that I was fat.

For far too many years I would put on and take off anywhere for 10-15 pounds it was a continuous up and down weight battles. However, since I met my husband Sean I gained 37 pounds in our first seven years of marriage and I had been trying to take it off unsuccessfully.

The opportunity to donate a kidney was really a great motivator to get the weight off. That is how I came up with the Ten – Nine – Twenty One, Forty Day Challenge. Now that I've lost the weight, it is just as important to maintain that success. The kidney transplant doctors emphasize the importance that I keep my weight under control after the surgery. This will be a lifelong challenge to maintain the positive eating habits I've developed on the Ten – Nine – Twenty One; Forty Day Challenge and to keep my BMI where it is now or lower.

1

For too many years I have been so obsessed with my weight. I knew it was time to start focusing less on what I weighted and start making wiser food choices. I have made the resolution that we're made to consume food, food was never meant to control us. 1 Corinthians 10:31 tells us, "*So, whether you eat or drink, or whatever you do, do everything to the glory of God.*"

Since the kidney surgery was about to happen in a few months I had to make a decision to really make a change in my eating habits. So I started by eating mostly green foods, fruits, vegetable and fish. I knew it was time to give up foods that triggered my unhealthy eating habits, so I gave up deserts first. I quickly noticed that I had more energy and just felt better. In Genesis 1:29, God said, "*I am giving you all the grain bearing plants and all the fruit trees. These trees make fruit with seeds in it. This grain and fruit will be your food.*"

Since my body was reacting poorly to certain foods. I decided to give up sugar, dairy, red meats, and anything with glutens in them. Since I removed these foods from my diet I have noticed a physical and emotional improvement in my body. I am no longer bloated or inflamed. I can think clearer, and it has helped me to lose weight and keep it off.

We don't get healthy accidental. It takes a deliberate effort, it's a choice, and it requires a lifestyle change. But it begins with a declaration. For long time success, a lifestyle change is a must if you are overweight and you won't change until you choose to change. It takes more than desire to get healthy it takes a decision. Everyone wants to be healthy, but very few people choose to be healthy. Long time success requires making wise choices. Then once you lose the weight to maintain your desired weight you must stick to new eating habits. Ephesians 4:22 tells us, *"You were told that your foolish desires will destroy you and that you must give up your old way of life with all its bad habits."*

If you have been stuck in a vicious cycle of defeat; it's time to follow God's directions into the Promised Land of freedom from food addiction. Deuteronomy 2:3 tells us, *"You have traveled around these mountains long enough. Turn north."* I also realize that my food choices matter to God and I am accountable for how I treat my body that is another reason I choose to make healthy eating habits. Romans 14:12 tells us, *"Each of us will give an account of ourselves to God."*

The simple facts about weight gain or loss is if we consume more calories than we burn up in exercise, we will gain weight and if we burn up more calories in exercise than we consume in food then we will reduce our weight. The weigh is always easier to put on than it is to get off. A lifestyle change requires a new ways of thinking. If we want to change how we act, we must begin by changing the way we think and talk. The way we think and talk controls the way we feel and the way we feel controls our actions. That is why a lifestyle change requires God's help.

The Holy Spirit can and will helps us break free from bad habits, compulsion eating, and food addictions when we ask Him for His guidance and help. We need to ask Jesus to give us knowledge and strength to keep our bodies strong and healthy. Then we will have no need to ask Him to heal a sick and diseased body that we created ourselves by not taking care of the Holy Spirit's temple.

I knew if I wanted to transform both my physical and spiritual health, I would need to come up with a healthy eating program. I was going to have to go to Scriptures and develop my own program based on God's Words. I realized if I wanted to eat healthy and not once again find myself in battle of defeat, it was time to replace food with Jesus. This time I am not losing weight for me but to honor the body God has given me.

Our habits are important if we want to accomplish victory. Because our habits governor our lives. Exchanging poor eating habits for healthy eating habits are essential for a permanent lifestyle change. Since our habits have been established over a long period of time. Changing them will take some hard work. Remember weight loss is by no means simple or quick. Those bad eating habits are a way of life. To change a habit we need to cultivate a whole new pattern of thinking. It is only through the strength of Jesus that I found victory. Psalm 28:7 tells us, *"The Lord is my strength and shield. I trusted Him with all my heart He helped me."*

Maintaining a healthy weight is a daily process. I wake up every morning with a choice to honor God with my body that day or not. Each choice I make determines my victory or defeat. It has to become a lifestyle change that is meant

4

to be carried on every day. For it to work it is going to take a complete dependence on Jesus. I realized that learning to hunger for Jesus instead of food, has abundant benefits and the way I care for my body is a part of my witness daily. Philippians 4:1 tells us, *"Christ is the one who gives me the strength I need to do whatever I must do."* I am confident that I can defeat this struggle through the strength that Jesus gives me. With the Holy Spirit guiding my every choice I will continue my journey to where there will be a healthier leaner me.

For a long time I knew that I had an eating issue. I have tried many different diet and read countless books on the subject of dieting. I have fasted with my church on a 21 day fast since 2000. Many years I extended the fast to 40 days. Even though by the end of the fast I was lighter, as soon as I started eating again, I put the weight back on and many years a few pounds more.

I ask Jesus daily to be my portion, strength, patience and wisdom. He has shown me that every day I need to lay down the strongholds that bound me for so long and I need to take hold of His promises. God's Word has opened my eyes and more importantly my heart to the truths I desperately needed to hear to become free of my food struggles. This entire journey has led me to be stronger and close to the Lord. I know that success can be a reality when Jesus is a part of it for that reason, He must be the in center of this life time journey, for victory to be mine.

There is victory in Jesus!

Fasting and Prayer

Through fasting and prayer we achieves a powerful means to draw closer to Jesus and we learn how to satisfy our desires for Jesus instead of food. He will encourage us when we want to eat unhealthy food choices. Do not rush into your fast make a promise to yourself and to God ahead of time. Write down what you plan on eating and omitting. If you have health concerns that need consideration check with your doctor before going on any fast.

Fasting is doing without foods that we do not really need or foods that has a control over our life. In addition, fasting does not mean that we should deprive yourselves of nutrition. As you fast you are applying self-control by turn down unhealthy food you once enjoyed or thought that you needed. While you are fasting, ask Jesus to satisfy your hunger and give you the desire to be healthy. Use your hunger as a motivation to pray instead of picking up a chip or a cookie. When we make prayer a habit before we put unhealthy food in our mouth the Holy Spirit will give us the desire and self-discipline to escape the urge. Ask the Holy Spirit to encourage you to find fulfillment in nutritious food choices. Matthew 5:6 tells us, "*Blessed are those who hunger and thirst for righteousness, for they shall be satisfied.*"

Fasting and Detoxification

A change of diet can be the first step to a healthier lifestyle. Fasting to lose weight might be the push that is needed to get your diet started. Fasting triggers detoxification; a healing process which allows the body to naturally cleanse itself. An unhealthy diet that's high in fat, sugars, and processed foods lets harmful bacteria accumulate which slows down the digestive systems.

Fasting with a well-balanced whole food vegetarian diet can help cleanse the body and can eventually eliminate many of the harmful effects of toxic foods. When we begin eating a more healthy vegetarian diet, we start to get more dietary fiber into our systems and our digestive systems start to work as it should. In addition, the dietary fiber found in whole foods, such as fruits, vegetables, nuts, and legume helps fill you up and keeps you feeling full longer so you eat less.

Ten – Nine – Twenty One

Chapter 2

Forty Day Challenge Program

I am thrilled you want to be healthier and I hope you will join me on the forty day challenge of permanent weight loss. The cleansing program that I have created has three parts and it is a forty day fast. This program is unique because it offers the benefits of fasting, but without totally going without food and nourishment. The first parts is an easy detox cleanse and the second and third parts are partial fasts that are fairly easy to follow, which makes it perfect for anyone who has never tried fasting before.

The first part of the detox cleanse program begins with a liquid fast of spicy lemon-limeade for the first ten days. The second part consist of a liquid fast on whole food with fresh fruit and vegetable juice, smoothies, pureed soups, and herbal tea for nine days. The third part is the Daniel fast with eating fruits, vegetables, legumes, nuts, seeds for twenty one days.

Ten Days

The first ten days consist of the spicy lemon-limeade cleanse. The spicy lemon-limeade cleanse rids our body of toxins that have built up over the years due to poor eating habits. It is one way of breaking the unhealthy eating cycle. Stanley Burroughs created the spicy lemonade fast also known as the Master Cleanse program in 1940 to cure stomach ulcer. Later in the year 1976, Stanley launched a book about it, stating that this cleansing program not only cures stomach ulcers, but also cleanses the colon, reduces

9

body weight, and also treats other disorders. According to Burroughs, toxins are caused by consuming meat, dairy, drugs, antibiotics, fungus-causing foods, pesticides and all the other junk that we put into our bodies. I totally agree with him.

On the ten day spicy lemon-limeade cleanse most people will see a large chunk of weight fall off. However, that's just starts the ball rolling; when you go off the cleanse you'll find you no longer desire unhealthy foods. Also, even though you will lose weight during the ten day cleanse, that isn't the goal. The goal is to purge your bodies of toxins and unhealthy eating habits that are weighing you down and start fresh.

In the first ten days of my cleanse I lose 10 lbs. It transform me in to a lighter, younger looking, and more energetic version of myself. I woke up every morning well rested and feeling better than the night before. The spicy lemon-limeade flushed out waste and restore my bodies so I was over flowing with energy. When I finish the spicy lemon-limeade fast not only did I crave healthier food, but I also was satisfied with smaller portions. I felt great because my body had been restored to a better state of health. I was delighted that I accomplished the first ten day feeling awesome.

The spicy lemon-limeade cleanse influence our bodies to crave healthy foods. Breaking unhealthy food addictions can be a very difficult that's why the spicy lemon-limeade cleanse is a great way to get started.

I did not experience any hunger on my ten day cleanse since I was getting an adequate amount of calories daily, enough to fuel my body for the day. The objective isn't to starve ourselves skinny, the objective is to flush the toxins out and get healthy. 1 tablespoon of grape B maple syrup has 55 calories. There are also 4 calories in each tablespoon of lemon juice, 8 calories in each drink. If you use 2 tablespoons of the maple syrup in each drinks and you are drinking 8 glasses a day that provides a daily calorie intake of 944 calories or if you are drinking 12 glasses a day that provides a daily calorie intake of 1,416.

The spicy lemon-limeade only has four ingredients and is easy to prepare. Grade B maple syrup, organic lemons and/or limes, cayenne pepper, and filtered water.

Grade B Maple Syrup - Grade B maple syrup is the most minimally processed of the maple syrups, making it more nutrient-dense. Grade B maple syrup also boosts your energy levels.

Cayenne Pepper - Cayenne pepper is a very good source of vitamins. Cayenne is a known to stimulate our body's circulation and reduces acidity. It helps decrease appetite and slows the growth of fat cells. Cayenne is great metabolic-booster, aiding the body in burning excess amounts of fats.

Lemon Juice - Lemon juice has Vitamin C in which helps to neutralize free radicals. Lemons are alkaline-forming on body fluids helping to restore balance to the body's ph. Lemons help produce bowel movements thus eliminating waste.

Lime Juice - Lime juice is rich in vitamin C and flavonoids a wonderful source of antioxidants which reduce the number of free radicals as well as detoxifies the body. Lime juice is also excellent weight reducer. In addition limes are good for digestion they have a mouthwatering scent that supports digestion.

Spicy Lemon-limeade Ingredients

Keep in mind that it is extremely important that you use only organic ingredients and don't make any substitution from the ingredients listed below. Make one glass at the time and always use freshly squeezed lemon and/or lime juice, then add the grade B maple syrup, cayenne pepper and filtered water, mix and drink immediately. Keep in mind the longer your spicy lemon-limeade sits, the more enzymes are lost. You should drink a minimum of 64 oz. 8- 8 oz. glasses of spicy lemon-limeade each day, but you can drink up to 12 glasses a day.

The lemon-limeade drink consists of:
2 tablespoons of fresh squeezed lemon and/or lime juice
2 tablespoons of organic grade B maple syrup
1/8 teaspoon cayenne pepper powder
8 ounces of filtered water

Herbal Laxative Teas

Bowel movements are essential to flush out the waste. So it is important to drink a cup of herbal laxative tea the night before you start your cleanse and every night that you are on the cleanse.

Nine Days

Whole Food Fruit and Vegetable Fast

The next nine days consist of a partial liquid fast with whole fruit and vegetable. A whole food liquid fast is an excellent way to continue the weight loss detox and cleansing processes after finishing the spicy lemon-limeade cleanse. A liquid fast is consuming foods that are in a liquid state as a sources of nutrition while excluding any solid foods. Food consumed during a liquid fast may include whole fruit and vegetable smoothies, fresh squeezed juices, whole vegetable pureed soups, herbal tea, and plenty of water. Liquid fasts are easier on your digestion system than solid foods.

It is possible to get the nutrition you need while consuming a liquid fast and you can continue to stay on this fast for long periods of time. The nutrients in whole food juices will provide energy and support your body while speeding up the detoxification process and releasing waste from your systems. Incorporating whole food juice as part of a balanced diet is a convenient way to add additional nutrition to your diet; than ordinary juicing because it contains more of the pulp and protein our bodies require. A serving or two of whole food juice usually meets the daily recommended intake of fruits and vegetables.

Whole Juice Recipe

Use a good high speed blender. Start by adding the liquid to your blender, followed by the soft fruit, add the greens or harder ingredients last. Blend on high for 90 seconds or until creamy.

Kale Pineapple Ginger
1/2 cup pineapple
1 large cucumbers
1 cup kale
1/2 lemon, squeezed
1/4 inch of ginger
1 cup filtered water

Kale Grapefruit
1 fresh squeezed grapefruit
1 cup kale
1 small apples
1/2 cup pineapple, cubed
1/2 cup of filtered water

Pineapple Spinach
1 cup pineapple, cubed
1 cup fresh spinach
1/4 cup fresh parsley
1 cup of filtered water

Black and Blueberry Banana
1 cup blueberries
1 cup blackberries
1 bananas
1 stalk celery
2 cups spinach
1 cup filtered water

Blackberries pineapple

1 cup blackberries

1 cups of pineapple

1 cup water, coconut milk, or almond milk

Peaches and Cream

1 cup peaches

1 cup coconut milk or almond milk

1 tsp freshly grated ginger

Tropical Fruit

1/2 mango, peeled and pitted

1/2 cup papaya

1 small banana

1/2 cup pineapple

1 cup of filtered water

Orange Cream

1 large frozen banana

1/2 tsp. vanilla extract

1 fresh orange rind removed

1 cup coconut milk or almond milk

Soup Recipes

Orange Ginger Carrot Soup

1 lb. bag of baby carrots

Juice from 2 oranges

1 inch piece of fresh ginger

2 cups vegetable broth

Place carrots in a pot with vegetable broth bring to boil, then simmer until tender. Let cool slightly. Pour carrots and

15

broth in to high speed blender add ginger and orange juice. Puree until soup has a smooth consistency Serve warm.

Cauliflower Soup
1 tablespoon coconut oil
1 clove garlic, crushed
1/4 teaspoon ground nutmeg
1/4 teaspoon freshly ground black pepper
1 1/2 teaspoons sea salt
6 cups water
1 head cauliflower, chopped
1/3 cup chopped sweep onion

In a large pot over medium heat, melt coconut oil add garlic, nutmeg, pepper and salt and pepper cook for 30 seconds, Pour in the water add cauliflower. Bring to a boil, then reduce heat, cover and simmer 20 minutes, until cauliflower is tender. Pour cauliflower and broth in to high speed blender. Puree until soup has a smooth consistency Serve warm.

Twenty One Days

Now you are ready to transition back to solid foods. The next twenty one days you will be eating a Daniel fast. It is a very healthy way to eat. The Daniel fast is a partial fast that is based on a vegetarian diet. Transitioning in to the Daniel fast will help you learn healthy eating habits that will make it easier to keep your weight down.

Daniel was a prophet in the Old Testament. The Daniel fast is a partial fast of plant-based nutrition. The first time we hear about the Daniel fast in the Bible was a ten day fast mentioned in the first chapter of Daniel. Daniel did not want to eat the king's rich food and wine because according to Jewish tradition it would make him unclean. Daniel 1:12 tells us, *"He said, Please give us this test for ten days. Don't give us anything but vegetables to eat and water to drink."*

The second time we hear about the Daniel fast was a twenty one day fast mentioned in the tenth chapter of Daniel. Daniel had a vision, the message was true and one of great conflict, and he understood the message and had understanding of the vision. Daniel 10:2 tells us, *"In those days I, Daniel, was mourning three full weeks."*

On a Daniel fast, you may eat a wide variety of whole foods including fruits, vegetables, root vegetables, dried legumes, nuts, seeds, fresh juices, whole juice smoothies, 100 percent pure fruit or vegetable juice, herbal tea and plenty of water. Keep in mind you are on a fast so limit yourself to only three meals a day and avoid over-eating and snacking.

Eating vegetables help improve your weight-loss progress. This is because many vegetables are high in fiber and low in calories, making them good choices for people who are trying to lose weight. Also people who get more fiber through their diet usually weigh less and have less body fat than people who don't eat enough fiber-rich foods.

There are two types of vegetables starchy and non-starchy. Both types are part of a proper diet. However, non-starchy varieties can be eaten in abundance. While starchy vegetables contain more sugar, calories, and carbohydrates therefore, portion size needs to be small and not eaten that often. Starchy vegetables include corn, peas, plantains, potatoes, squash, beans, beets, carrots, pumpkins, and yams.

Fruits and berries are a key part of a healthy diet especially if you are trying to lose weight; without adding any unnecessary fats. They provide the energy and nearly every nutrient that our body needs to reduce weight. Fruits provide nutrients necessary for good health and maintenance of our body. They benefit our body greatly as they provide a natural sources of vitamins and minerals, which are essential for the proper functioning of the body. Eating fruit is a great way to get a range of antioxidant, vitamins, minerals, folic acid, and potassium. In addition fruit is a healthy carbohydrate food because it is alkaline forming and they are naturally low in sodium. They are rich in dietary fiber they contains soluble and insoluble fiber, which helps keep our colon free of toxins and also help to improve the functioning of the digestive tract.

Fruit makes an excellent and satisfying snack. Eating a piece of fruit can satisfy a sweet craving without any detrimental effects. Fruit is filling because it's filled with fiber and water, many fruits have up to 90% water. That makes them an awesome weight loss food. Eating an apple 30 minutes before a meal will fill you up and prevent you from overeating. Fruits are naturally low in fat, sodium, calories, and they are cholesterol free.

Legumes can be eaten on your weight-loss program they are packed with essential nutrients. Legumes fits into the protein food group, since they are rich in protein. They are also very high in fiber. In addition, beans help keep you feeling full longer. Which can help you lose weight when eaten in recommended portions. Keep in mind beans are not low in calories and can lead to weight gain when consumed in excess.

Nuts and seeds are also high in protein and an excellent source of healthy oils like omega 3. Although, nuts and seeds are a healthy snack because they are high in oils, and carbohydrates, you only need a small handful of them to get a serving from the protein group. Calories can add up quickly and pounds will come back on if you eat too many nuts and seeds.

You can also include healthy oils, spices, herbs, stevia, and, vinegar when preparing your food. There are many benefits from cooking with herbs and spices. Adding herbs and spices to your food gives your meals extra flavor, and you also get health benefits because herbs and spices contain antioxidants, minerals, and vitamins. In addition some herbs and spices can help you maintain a healthy body weight by promoting weight loss. So be very generous when adding spices to your food.

Things Not to Include in Part Three

While on the twenty one day Daniel fast you are leave out all meat and animal products including beef, veal, pork, bacon, ham, chicken, duck, lamb, venison, mutton, seafood and fish, all dairy products, including cheese, cream, butter, eggs, sweeteners, sugar, honey, syrups, molasses, and cane juice. As well as, refined and processed food, artificial flavorings, food additives, chemicals, foods that contain artificial preservatives. Deep fried foods, shortening, margarine, and foods high in fat.

Some Daniel fast plans include grains however, we will be omitting them for the next twenty one days. Since one of the goals on these programs is to lose weight. Then we will slowing introducing them back in to our diets. That said, omit all bread , baked goods, pastries, cookies, cakes, all grains, including but not limited to all wheat, rye, barley, brown rice, millet, quinoa, oats, barley, grits, all pasta, rice cakes, popcorn, corn and flour tortillas.

Psalm 104:14 tells us, *"He causes the grass to grow for the cattle, and herb for the service of man: that he may bring forth food out of the earth."*

Vegetable Recipes

15 Bean Soup
1 - 1 lbs. package of 15 dried b bean
4 cups vegetable broth
1 tablespoon olive oil
1 large onion, chopped
1 garlic clove, chopped
2 celery stalks thinly sliced
2 carrots, thinly sliced
1 cup diced tomatoes
8 tablespoons lemon juice
1 tablespoon oregano

2 teaspoons ground thyme
1 teaspoon cayenne pepper
½ tablespoon ground black pepper
½ tablespoon salt

Soak beans overnight, or at least 8 hours. Drain and rinse. In a 2 quart pot cook beans in 2 quarts of water until slightly tender by simmering on the stove for about 1 1/2 hours. Shortly before the beans are done, sauté onion, garlic, oregano, ground thyme in oil until slightly brown. When beans are done, drain half the cooking water. Add all remaining ingredients and simmer, uncovered, for 40-60 minutes, stirring occasionally. Adjust seasoning to taste.

Cucumber Basil Salad
1 large red onion, minced
2 cups fresh baby spinach, finely chopped
3 tablespoons chopped fresh basil, finely chopped
1 pound tomatoes, minced
2 large seedless cucumbers, peeled and minced

Place above ingredient in large bowl with an air-tight lid and refrigerate salad, overnight.

Basil Dressing
1/4 cup red wine vinegar
2 tablespoons extra virgin olive oil
1   garlic clove, minced
1 teaspoon sea salt
1 teaspoon cracked black pepper

Drizzle over salad, let stand 10 minutes before serving.

Asian Coleslaw
5 cups thinly sliced green cabbage
2 cups thinly sliced red cabbage
2 cups shredded Napa cabbage
2 red bell peppers, thinly sliced
2 carrots, julienned
6 green onions, chopped
1/2 cup fresh cilantro chopped

Place above ingredient in large bowl

Dressing
6 tablespoons rice wine vinegar
6 tablespoons olive oil
5 tablespoons creamy peanut butter
3 tablespoons soy sauce
3 tablespoons brown sugar
2 tablespoons minced fresh ginger root
1 1/2 tablespoons minced garlic

In a small bowl, whisk the dressing ingredients together and pour the dressing over the salad. Toss until the salad is evenly coated with dressing.

Kale Salad
½ cup almonds, coarsely chop
8 ounces kale chopped
8 ounces red cabbage thinly sliced
½ cup dried cranberries
1 medium honey crisp apple, chopped into small pieces

Place above ingredient in large bowl

Dressing
3 tablespoons olive oil
1½ tablespoons apple cider vinegar
1 tablespoon smooth Dijon mustard
2 teaspoons stevia
Sea salt and freshly ground pepper, to taste

In a small bowl, whisk the dressing ingredients together and pour the dressing over the salad. Toss until the salad is evenly coated with dressing.

Ending the Fast

One of the most important phases of fasting is ending it correctly. How you break a fast is extremely important for your physical and spiritual well-being. That is why it is so important to end a fast gradually. Since our digestive system has gone without unhealthy and large quantities of food for forty days you may encounter reactions like an upset stomach and weight gain if you suddenly eat a full meal or unhealthy foods after ending a fast. Our bodies need time to adapt as we bring back foods we have avoided.

Begin slowly with smaller portions and little by little increase the quantity each day. Start with adding brown rice, black rice, wild rice, steel cut oats, quinoa, eggs, fish, and poultry. Keep in mind if you start eating the way you were before you lost the weight on the fast you will gain it back quickly. You have worked so hard to take the weight off so make a resolution to stay the course by carrying on the healthy eating habits you created on the fast. In

Genesis *1:29*, God said, *"I am giving you all the grain bearing plants and all the fruit trees. These trees make fruit with seeds in it. This grain and fruit will be your food."*

Terri Flynn

Ten – Nine – Twenty One

Chapter 3

Conclusion

Keep in mind that fasting should redirect our appetite from food to Jesus. Fasting helps us to see that Jesus is more pleasing than eating. When we allow our physical appetites to rule our life, and we can't imagine anything better than food, we are allowing food to become an idol. However, through fasting and prayer we begin to make Jesus the center of our life and we begin to see things in a different way. We begin to see food as a gifts from God. We begin to enjoy growing in fellowship with Jesus more than pleasing our appetite. Philippians 3:19 *"Their destination is destruction, their god is their appetite, their glory is in their shame, their minds are set on earthly things."*

Never fast for the sake of dieting; fast for the sake of God. Dieting and fasting both involve saying no to some foods, however, the goals are different. When we diet we seem to care more about our physical bodies than about the spiritual bodies. A diet limits food for physical reasons; but a fast limits food for spiritual reasons. Fasting is not just a self-improvement project. However, you will experience a healthier and leaner you at the end of this forty day challenge; that is a benefit not the end goal. Real fasting is turning attention away from ourselves and turning our attention to Jesus. For the next forty days start treating your body like God's temple, because it is God's temple. To learn more about Fasting read; *Fasting a Spiritual Discipline with Physical Benefits, Cleansing the Holy Spirit's Temple.*

About the Author

Terri Flynn was born and raised in Kingston, New York. At age 12 a seed was planted in her heart that would slowly grow and mature to a passionate love for Christ. In 1999, she surrendered her life to Jesus and began to seek after God through fasting, prayer, and meditating on His promises. It was through these times of prayer and study that Terri discovered that God's promises apply to the spiritua , emotional, physical, and financial areas of her life.

A desire for the Word of God was rooted in Terri's life when she was attended Spirit Vision Bible College; at which time she made a commitment to say yes to whatever God asked. She wholeheartedly believes in the Word of God ard has a passion for praying and proclaiming His promises. She has faith that God has made promises to us in His Word and as believers we should trust His promises. Terri discovered the power to live victoriously by applying God's Word to her life and wants to support others to do the same. She published her first book *God Delights in the Prayers of His Children*, in 2013.

Terri is active in her local church, Free Chapel, and she considers it a privilege to serve as a volunteer. She believes that the blessings and talents she has been given should be used to bless others. She has served in children's, youth, marriage, women's, and prayer ministries, as well as other outreach ministries. She also attended School of Discipleship, and Joy School of Ministry. She married Sean in 2007; they reside in Georgia with their blended family.

Enjoy this additional book from author Terri Flynn

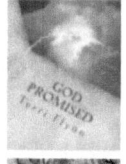 **God Delights in the Prayers of His Children**
Praying God's Word Back to Him through Scripture-Based Prayer

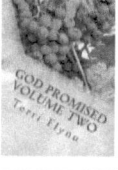 **Fasting a Spiritual Discipline with Physical Benefits**
Cleansing the Holy Spirit's Temple

God Promised
Proclaiming the Word Over

Volume One - Joy, Love, Faith, Peace, & Kindness

Volume Two - Worry, Anger, Fear, Anxiety, & Depression

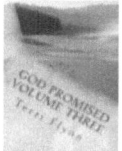 Volume Three -   Prayer, Fasting, Giving, Strength, & Finances

Available for purchase online and as e-book
(Prayer Book) https://www.createspace.com/5176418
(Fasting Book) https://www.createspace.com/5653724
(Volume 1) https://www.createspace.com/4926657
(Volume 2) https://www.createspace.com/5194452
(Volume 3) https://www.createspace.com/5213557
Visit me at: terriflynnauthor.weebly.com
https://www.facebook.com/PrayerRequestsTerriFlynn.org

www.ingramcontent.com/pod-product-compliance
Lightning Source LLC
Chambersburg PA
CBHW020906310526
45786CB00018B/1931